The Dougy Center for Grieving Children
3909 S.E. 52nd Avenue
P.O. Box 86852 Portland, OR 97286

Phone: 503-775-5683

Fax: 503-777-3097

Email: help@dougy.org

Website: www.dougy.org

Written and printed in the United States of America.

ISBN: 1-890534-03-x

Revised 7/2004, 9/2010

Our Mission

The mission of The Dougy Center for Grieving Children is to provide to families in Portland and the surrounding region loving support in a safe place where children, teens and their families grieving a death can share their experiences as they move through their healing process. Through our National Center for Grieving Children & Families we also provide support and training locally, nationally and internationally to individuals and organizations seeking to assist children in grief.

The Dougy Center is supported solely through private support from individuals, foundations and companies, and receives no state or federal funding. The Dougy Center does not charge a fee for its services.

Table of Contents

Development of this guidebook was
made possible through a grant from the
Meyer Memorial Trust

Introduction

How can I help a grieving child?

If you know a child who has experienced the death of a mother, father, caregiver, sister, brother or friend, you may have wondered how you can help. At The Dougy Center for Grieving Children, we have worked with thousands of grieving children and teens since our program began in 1982. They've taught us a lot about what does and does not help them. We also hear every day from caring parents, teachers and adult caregivers who want to support grieving children, but aren't sure how to go about it. In response to that concern, we've gathered together the most important stuff we've learned from the kids, and the result is this guidebook. The information in these pages is simple and practical and is drawn from the stories of children and teenagers who have been on the front lines of grief.

One of the most important things we've learned from children is that everyone grieves differently. Cultural traditions, religious beliefs, family experiences and personality differences all influence the way we choose to express our grief. Not all the suggestions in this guidebook will apply to your situation. Take what is useful and helpful for you. When in doubt, ask a child or teenager what helps. They will tell you.

1

Listen

After a death, many children want to share their story. They may want to tell you what happened, where they were when they were told about the death and what it was like for them. Telling their story is a healing experience. One of the best ways adults can help young grievers is to listen to their stories.

As adults, we're often too quick to offer advice, give opinions and make judgments. We think we know what's best for our children, and we want to make sure they get the right information. But while we're busy talking, we sometimes miss important messages from children about what they need and how we can best help them. Suggestions for being a good listener:

- Don't give advice or make judgments
- Reflect back what the child says using the child's words
- Paraphrase the child's words
- Ask clarifying questions

Here's an example of a child's statement and adult responses using the above suggestions:

Child— *"My daddy died in a plane crash. At first, I was sad. But then I was so angry when I found out they let him fly when it was a storm. I yelled at the guy from the airline. I hate him."*

Don't:
Give advice or make judgments:

Adult— *"Hate is a very strong word. You probably don't hate him. You're mad now, but you'll get over it. It's a horrible thing that happened."*

Do:
Reflect back what the child said using the child's words:

Adult— *"So your dad died in a plane crash. You felt sad at first, but then you were angry because they let him fly when the weather was stormy. So you yelled at the guy at the airline, and you feel that you hate him."*

Paraphrase the child's words:

Adult— *"It sounds like you felt many different feelings after your dad died. Sad feelings. Mad feelings and feelings of hate."*

Ask clarifying questions:
"So what was it like when you felt all those different feelings?"
"So what kinds of things do you do when you feel sad? Or angry?"

Go to the Hostpital.

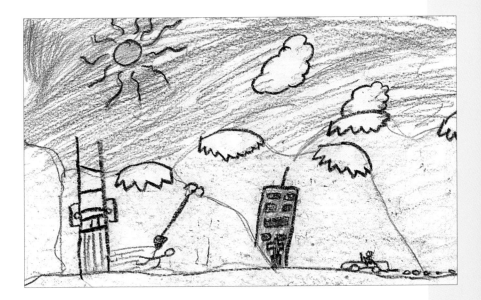

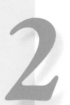

Listen some more

Sometimes, children don't want to talk, or can't find the words. Or, they protect the adults around them from more pain. Some kids just aren't verbal. When you listen, pay attention to what they're not saying, as well. They will often reveal a lot about what's going on through their actions and not just their words. Once they believe you can be trusted, they may begin to open up to you, sharing their thoughts and emotions.

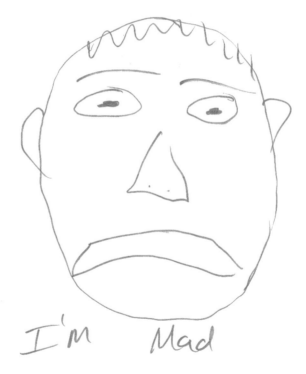

I'M Mad

Be honest. Never lie to a child

Let's face it. It's hard to tell kids painful things because we want to protect them from pain. That's part of our "job" as adults. When we have to break the news and details about a death, it's natural to want to protect children, as if we can somehow cushion the blow by not telling the whole story. Sometimes, we don't want to tell children the truth because we want to protect them from possible harsh realities about a death—like the extent of someone's physical suffering before death, the details of a murder, the reality of a suicide.

But the truth is, whether we tell them directly or not, children usually learn the facts in one way or another, either by overhearing adults or other kids talking, or, in some cases, from television or newspapers. It only complicates a child's grief when someone close lies about the cause of death and the deceased. It also sends a message that it's okay to hide the truth, and that adults are not to be trusted. One way adults hide the truth is by talking around sensitive topics. But even preschoolers catch onto this game. They are able to sense that something is wrong, and notice when adults act differently.

For three days, no one talked to 9-year-old Betty about the fact that her mom, who was missing, was probably dead. All the adults around her talked very quietly and sent her out to play when they wanted to talk. On the fourth day, her father told her that her mother had drowned. Betty was very angry with her father and other relatives for not sharing with her what they knew. She asked her father, "Why wasn't it important enough to tell me?"

3

4 Answer the questions they ask. Even the hard ones

Kids learn by asking questions. When they ask questions about a death, it's usually a sign that they're curious about something they don't understand. After his dad died of stomach cancer, Brad, 8, was very curious about the illness. When he attended support groups at The Dougy Center, he met other children who had experienced cancer deaths. Week after week, he asked the other children questions: "What kind of cancer?" or "What was it like?" Often, he started group conversations about what cancer is from a child's perspective, and what it's like for a child to live with someone who is dying from cancer. Through his questions, Brad connected with other children who could understand his experience, which led him to the discovery that he was not alone in his struggles.

"Cancer is something that gets in your cells, and it makes you tired, and you get thin, and somebody has to take care of you."

—*Jenny, 10*

As an adult, one of the most important things you can do for children is to let them know that all questions are okay to ask, and to answer their questions truthfully. Be sensitive to their age and the language they use. Children don't want to hear a clinical, adult-sounding answer to their questions, but they don't want to be lied to either. Often, the hardest time to be direct is right after a death. When a child asks what happened, use concrete words such as "died" or "killed," instead of vague terms like "passed away." A young child who hears his mother say, "Dad passed away," or, "I lost my husband," may expect that his father will return or simply needs to be found.

If you don't know the answer to a child's question, it's acceptable to say "I don't know." If you can find the answer, do so and get back to the child with the answer. Some questions may not have an answer, such as, "Why did Mom kill herself?"

Give the child choices whenever possible

Children appreciate having choices as much as adults do. They have opinions, and feel valued when allowed to choose. And they don't like to be left out. For example, it is a meaningful and important experience for children to have the opportunity to say goodbye to the person who died in a way that feels right to them. They can be included in the selection of a casket, clothing, flowers and the service itself. Some children may also want to speak or write something to be included in the service, or to participate in some other way.

After a death, having choices allows children to grieve a death in the way that is right for them. Sometimes, children in the same family will choose differently. For example, one child may want pictures and memorabilia of the person who died, while another may feel uncomfortable with too many reminders around. If you are a parent, ask your children what feels right to them. Don't assume that what holds true for one child will be the same for another.

Allowing choices also provides another benefit for grieving children: it helps them regain some of the sense of control they have lost after the death.

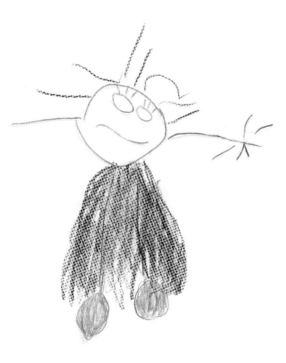

6 Encourage consistency and routines

When a death occurs, it pulls the rug out from under a child. Life feels chaotic, unsafe and unpredictable. You can help rebuild a sense of stability for a child by providing consistency and routines. Accomplishing small tasks and returning to daily routines helps alleviate the sense of disorder and anxiety that naturally accompanies a loss. Routines also create a sense of continuity between life before the death and afterwards.

If you are a parent, you know that a death in the family is often followed by many changes, some of which may be unexpected and add an extra element of stress to your life. Perhaps your family's financial situation has changed, and/or you have to move to another city or home. Children may have to leave schools and friends and take on new roles and responsibilities in the family.

Sometimes, we forget that each change is another loss. Often, changes intensify the already difficult grief experience. Too many changes put pressure on children, and some may find it difficult to adjust. As you make the necessary adjustments to your life following a death, you can help your children by maintaining consistency in certain routines in their lives, such as bedtimes, mealtimes and family times. Even though activities will be different without the presence of the deceased, children will feel added safety and security from knowing that they can count on some routines to continue after the death.

Mealtimes can be especially difficult for grieving families; the absence of the person who died is so painfully obvious. As painful as they can be, family meals can have a significant stabilizing effect on children.

"Since my mom died, we go out every night. I just wish we could eat at home. I'm tired of never being at home. My dad seems to be running away from some ghost."

—*Kevin, 11*

Talk about and remember the person who died

Remembering a person who died is part of the healing process. One way to remember is simply to talk about the person who died. It's okay to use his or her name and to share what you remember about that person. You might say, "Your dad really liked this song," or, "Your mom was the best pie maker I know."

Bringing up the name of the person who died is one way to give children permission to share their feelings about the deceased. It reminds them that it is not "taboo" to talk about the deceased. Sharing a memory has a similar effect. It also reminds the child that the person who died will continue to "live on" and impact the lives of those left behind.

"My daddy tickled me. He danced with me. He read to me."

—Sarah, 9

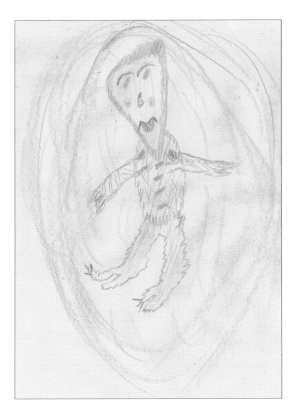

At The Dougy Center, children often bring memorabilia from the deceased, such as pictures, possessions, poems and memories, to share with other children. Sometimes, they light candles in memory of the person who died.

Children also like to have keepsakes of the person who died. Usually, they are interested in objects which hold an emotional or relational significance. When his father died of a heart attack, Jeremy, 12, asked if he could have his work boots. Although they were old, worn out and too big for his feet, they served as a memory of all the times his father had taken him to the construction site where he worked. Tom, 16, wanted to keep his dad's flannel shirt. When they went fishing, his dad always wore that shirt; now Tom wears it when he goes fishing.

"I remember my dad because he was always there for me."

—Nicole, 12

When possible, children should be given choices about what possessions and photos to keep. One way to do this is to invite children and teens to participate in the process of sorting, keeping and discarding the possessions of the person who died. Additionally, this serves as a concrete way for children to say "goodbye." If a child chooses not to participate or is too young, we suggest that some items be stored for the child to have later.

"We planted columbines because those were my mom's favorite flower. When I see them, I think of her in the garden."

—Jeannie, 11

Make a child's world safe for grieving

There aren't a lot of places where children are encouraged to talk openly about death and mourning. Sometimes, it's up to adult caregivers—parents, relatives, teachers, friends—to help children find places where it is not only permissible, but encouraged, to express their grief. Children need trusted support people in their lives to turn to after a death. In addition to their parents, some may seek out a teacher, relative or family friend.

Some kids feel isolated from their friends after a death because they view themselves as different from their peers. It may be difficult to identify supportive people at first because some friends may be comfortable talking about grief while others may not. A peer support group is often an effective way of connecting grieving children with other kids their age. Others may find counseling helpful. What's important is that the child or teen knows he or she has at least one place to feel safe with his or her grief. If you are the parent of a grieving child, work with your child to make a list of persons or places to go to when he or she needs to talk or lean on the shoulder of a friend. It can also be helpful to identify families who have undergone similar experiences.

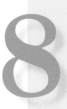

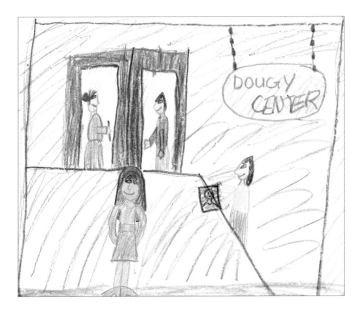

Expect and allow all kinds of emotions. Shocked, sad, numb, mad, glad…

When 15-year-old Ray's mother died after many months of being ill with leukemia, he felt relieved. "I was relieved because she wasn't suffering and in pain any more."

Sadie, 12, whose mother died of alcoholism, said she couldn't feel sad her mother died because of her drinking problem.

Feelings and grief reactions are influenced by all sorts of things: the type of death, the age of the child, and the nature of the relationship the child shared with the person who died.

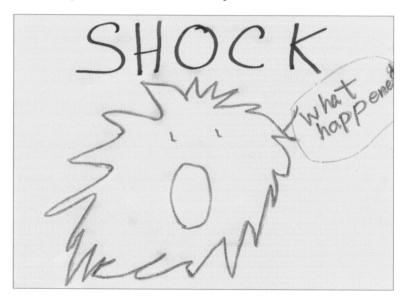

Allow for any and all emotions in your children—anger, frustration, embarrassment. As parents or adult caregivers, you can help a child feel safe by listening to and not putting down his or her feelings. Validating emotions will also help the child recognize that it's acceptable to feel a wide variety of emotions, and to allow each one to express feelings in a safe manner. If a child is angry and feels like hitting something, you might encourage him or her to express angry feelings with pillows, a punching bag or stuffed animals, rather than saying, "You shouldn't be mad."

Forget about the "grief stages"

Some people say grief follows a linear course of sequential stages. You may have heard about them: denial, anger, bargaining, depression, acceptance. The families we've worked with tell a different story. Grieving may include one, all or none of the so-called stages, and not in any particular order. Also, grief does not have a particular endpoint. As one young Dougy Center participant put it: "People may tell you you're supposed to be done with your grieving, but grief never ends." Sharon, a college student and volunteer at The Dougy Center, described her grieving as a series of waves, some of which are big and stormy, and others calm.

While you can expect children to eventually return to a normal level of functioning and to enjoy life, don't expect them to wrap up or graduate from their grief. Or, if by chance they seem to be recovering and reintegrating into life faster than you are, don't worry. They may just be riding another wave.

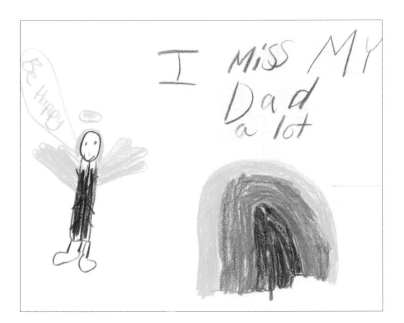

11 Respect differences in grieving styles

For 8-year-old Jolie, whose mother died of a heart attack, grieving was a series of crying jags, one after another. In the days and weeks after her mother died, tears and talking helped soothe the pain. Meg, Jolie's teenage sister, never shed a tear and showed little emotion when the topic of her mother came up. Meg said she liked to keep busy and felt better when she was shooting baskets and spending time with her friends. This was all very confusing to the girls' stepfather, who concluded that Meg wasn't grieving because she hadn't cried and she hadn't talked much about her mother. In fact, Jolie's and Meg's responses to their mother's death were both typical. Children's grieving styles—even in the same family—can be completely opposite.

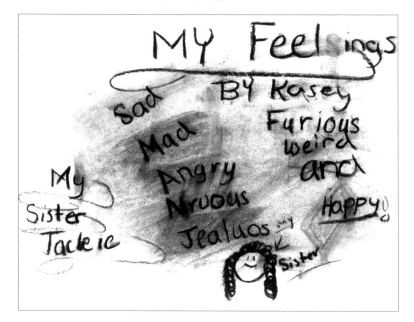

Recognizing that each person grieves in his or her own way is essential to the healing process for a family. Listen to children talk about their feelings and watch their behavior, and you will help clarify and affirm these natural differences.

Get out the crayons, pens, pencils, paint and chalk

Not all children are talkers, and not all grief emotions are easily expressed verbally. Artwork, poetry, journaling and other modes of creative expression are wonderful outlets for working through emotions and thoughts associated with the death or the deceased.

At The Dougy Center, children use artwork to memorialize and appreciate some aspect of the person who died. Here are a few ways to invite children or teens to express their grief:

- Provide paper, pencils, crayons, and felt pens for drawing
- Give the child or teen a grief journal to record thoughts and feelings
- Co-write a story with your teen or child about the person who died
- Get out paints and make a big painting
- Use clay for pounding and sculpting
- Collect magazines and make a collage
- Create a family tree

Molly, 6, missed her daddy very much after he died. So every day at school she drew a picture of him and kept it on her desk to have him with her while she worked.

"My aunt really helped me. We put up a huge piece of butcher paper and started drawing my dad's family tree. We did a little every day. Talking about my dad and his family really helped."

—*Katie, 13*

Morgan, 10, created a memory box from a shoe box which he covered with pictures of his mom. Now, whenever he draws pictures or writes a memory of his mom he puts it in his special memory box and can look at the things he has collected.

Alice, 8, made a clay grave marker after her dad died. It had his date of death and a quotation she loved. She has it in her room because her dad's grave is far away, and she does not get to go very often.

Mike, 18, made a diploma from clay for his mom, who had died and would never get to see him graduate.

Ann, 11, made a mask of grief from clay. It showed her face as she really felt, not the face she showed the world.

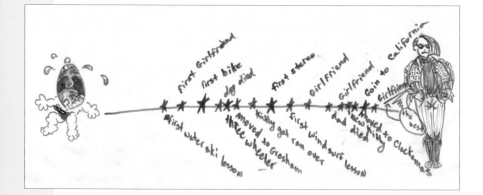

Run! Jump! Play! (Or find other ways to release energy and emotions)

13

After his father died of a heart attack, the kindest words 15-year-old Michael heard were not condolences. "The priest told me, 'When it gets to be too much, take a baseball bat and hit a tree,' " Michael recalled. "It sounded a little crazy at the time, but I was mad, and it worked."

Not everyone needs to hit a tree. But exercise and physical play do help children release energy and emotions. At The Dougy Center, children punch punching bags and stuffed animals, and have pillow fights in a room called the Volcano Room. We keep these activities safe with rules such as "No Head Shots" and "No Hitting People." Often, a child will choose to go to the Volcano Room after he or she has shared something difficult about the death with peers. A few other activities you might try are throwing Nerf balls, beating drums or tearing/crumpling paper. Other physical activities might include running, shooting hoops, kicking a soccer ball or dancing. All are good outlets for releasing energy and feelings.

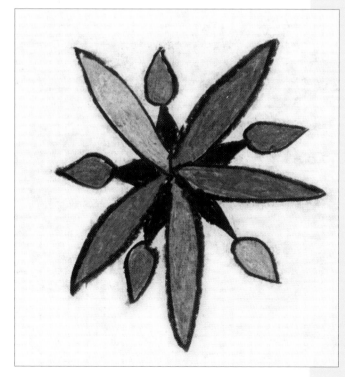

17

14

Be a model of good grief

Children watch adults to get cues about how they are "supposed" to grieve. They learn from watching and imitating the adults around them. Children look to their parents for cues about grieving—from how to talk about the death to what emotions are acceptable.

Parents who attend to their own grief processes in positive ways set a good example for their children. Sometimes, parents want to hide their grief from their children, thinking that it will upset them. Yet it's important for a child to know that it's acceptable to cry, to feel angry, to grieve. Children often will not show emotions because they don't want to upset the surviving parent or others.

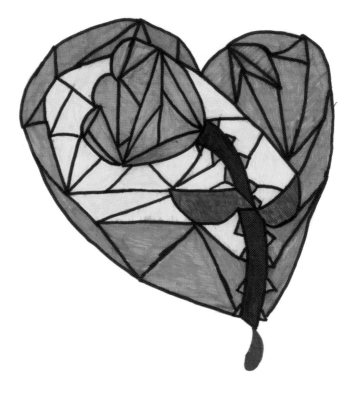

Hug with permission

Children need lots of assurance after a death, particularly if they have lost a parent. Many grieving children fear that they will lose the other parent and are anxious about separating from the surviving parent. As parents, you can help your child reestablish a sense of security and attachment to you through extra hugs and affection.

Bear in mind, though, that some kids don't like to be hugged. If you're trying to comfort a child, be sure to ask if it's okay to hug him or her. It's important that we don't impose our own needs for affection on the child.

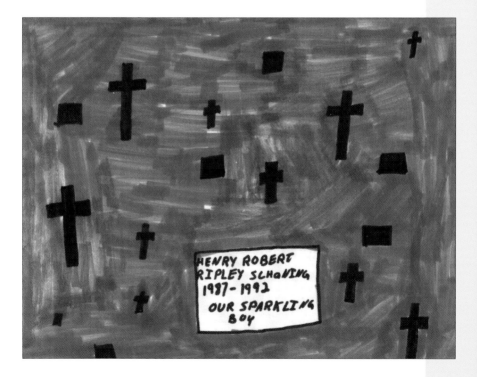

16 Practice patience

If you are a grieving parent, you've probably noticed that there are up days and down days. Days when you are on the ball, and days when you feel you are functioning about as well as a slug. Kids go through this, too. Sometimes, they find it hard to concentrate on schoolwork. They get frustrated and want a break. Grieving children are often clumsy with their hands and feet, spilling liquids and stumbling. Be patient with children—and yourself—on down days.

In the first few months after their father died in a boating accident, the Jones family made an agreement about taking time out on hard days. Occasionally, Jessica, 8, or James, 12, needed to take a day off and spend some time resting. Sometimes, Mom took the kids out of school for the day. As a family, they went to the park to play or to have lunch at their favorite restaurant, where they went with their dad before he died.

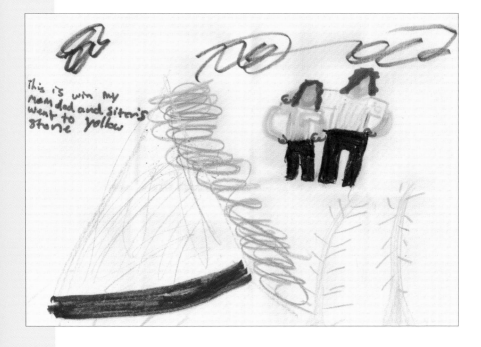

This is win my mom dad and siters went to yollow stone

Support children even when they are in a bad mood

No one likes being in a bad mood, or being around others who are. When you're grieving, bad moods seem to appear suddenly, like little dark clouds camped above your head. How did they get there, you wonder, and when will they go away? It's hard to tell. Grieving children slip into bad moods just as adults do. Sometimes, something may remind the child of the person who died. Or, the child may feel frustrated that nothing is the same since Dad died.

Ned, 12, said he felt grouchy whenever he thought about the mystery of his mom's death. No one knew if it was an accident or suicide. In some children, an irritable mood is like a mask for sadness that is too hard to express.

On the other hand, kids often have no idea why they're in a funk. As an adult, it's possible to support and empathize with a child's bad mood without figuring it out or fixing it. While honoring the child's mood, it may also help to invite the child to participate in activities he or she has always enjoyed.

Remember to validate the child's feelings first, then encourage good choices. Children need to know that it's normal and natural to feel the way they do.

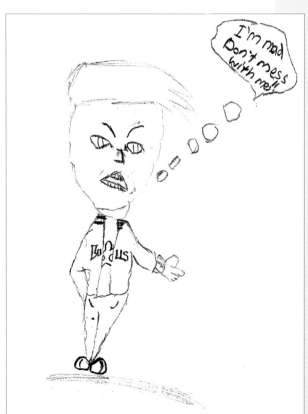

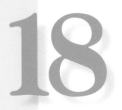

18 Expect some kids to act younger than their age

Kids often feel anxious and insecure after a death. Sometimes, they lapse into behaviors of younger children. Such behavior is not unusual. For example, a young child may want to sleep in his parent's bed.

Others may wet their own bed, throw tantrums or pick up habits they had as a younger child. When these behaviors occur, be supportive and understanding. Don't ridicule or punish the behavior, but allow it for a time. The child will return to his or her higher functioning when he or she is coping better in their grief. However, persistent and ongoing regressive behaviors should be checked by a medical professional.

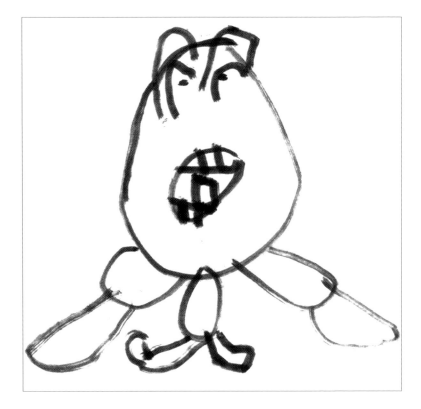

Expect some kids to become little adults

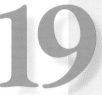

Some kids become hyper-responsible after a death. Sometimes, it's because they're acting out what people have told them: "You're the man of the house now," after a father's death. Or, "You'll have to take care of your dad," after a mother has died. Sometimes, they're working extra hard not to be a problem or burden to the surviving parent, or working extra hard to keep their pain at bay. You can help children or teens keep their childhood or youth by not allowing them to become miniature adults or surrogate parents. Children or teens can become resentful and rebellious if they are forced to become a "mother" or "father" to younger siblings.

After her mother died, Mary, 14, was expected to take on the mother's role for her father and two younger brothers. Because she was the only girl in the house, and the only one who knew how to cook and clean, it was considered her role. She was happy to help out the family but found that she had no time for her own activities or friends.

Tom, 10, began helping with repairs, chores and decisions after his father died. When his father was alive, Tom often tagged along while his father made household repairs. It was a special time. For his 10th birthday, Tom asked his mother for a hammer and drill so he could do the repairs like his dad did. When his mother tried to do a repair, he said, "That's not the way Dad would do it." Even though his mother encouraged him to be a kid, Tom seemed to enjoy the role of helping out and being "the man of the house."

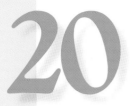

20 Encourage kids to eat right and drink lots of water

Changes in appetite are not uncommon after a death. Some kids find comfort in eating, while others lose their appetite. Whenever possible, encourage healthy eating. Unhealthy eating patterns (or too much junk food) may compound already difficult emotions and low energy after a death. Persistent ongoing changes in appetite or extreme weight fluctuation should be addressed by a medical professional.

Grieving is draining, literally. Children and adults get dehydrated as they exert physical and mental energy in the grief process. Drinking lots of water rehydrates cells and helps restore depleted energy. It is important to drink water and juices frequently, especially in the early stages of grieving.

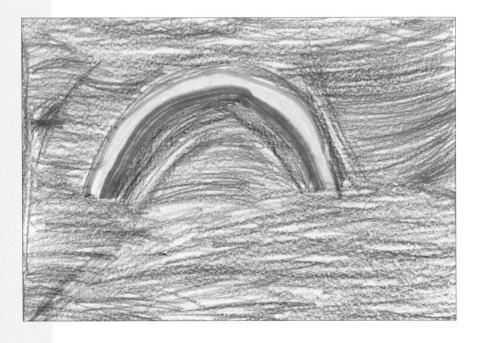

Help the child at bedtimes. Sleep may come hard for grieving children

Bedtimes are often tough after the death of a special person. If you are a parent, you may notice your child has difficulty separating from you, especially if the person who died was a parent. Your child may have nighttime fears, difficulty falling asleep, awakening early or nightmares. Bedtime is a time when activity ceases and thoughts may surface of the person who died. It can be difficult for a child to put these thoughts to rest.

One of the ways you can help is to have consistent bedtime rituals, such as a story, a song, conversation or prayers. These times together will help reestablish a child's sense of security and assure him or her that you are there when he or she needs you. Staying with the child until he or she falls asleep, or allowing him or her to sleep with you, is also an option.

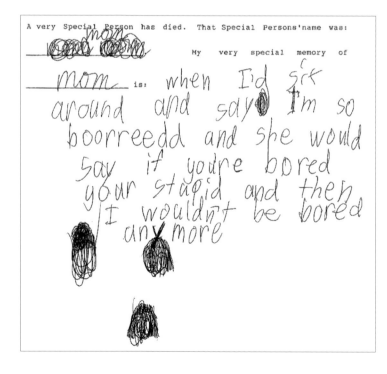

A very Special Person has died. That Special Persons'name was: _mom_

My very special memory of _mom_ is: when I'd sit around and saye I'm so boorreedd and she would say if youre bored your stupid and then I wouldn't be bored any more

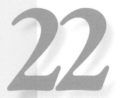

Inform the child's teacher about the death

Children spend a lot of time in school. A death impacts not only family life but also school life. That's why it's important to inform a child's teacher, counselor, coaches and any other close adult support person in the school setting about the death. Not all children will have difficulty going back to school. Some may even find refuge in schoolwork and activities. Others may have trouble concentrating and keeping up with their homework in the weeks and months following a death.

Sometimes, it's helpful to meet with a child's teacher and to develop a plan for completion of schoolwork. If you are a counselor or teacher and are working with a child who is struggling with schoolwork, you may want to set small reachable goals to help him or her regain confidence as he or she catches up and improves performance.

Some children may not want teachers and classmates to know about the death. Be sensitive to what the child wants shared and what she or he wants kept private.

For more information on helping the grieving student, see the resource section in the back of this guidebook.

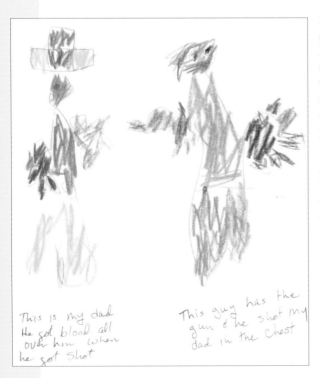

This is my dad
He got blood all
over him when
he got shot

This guy has the
gun & he shot my
dad in the chest

Resist being overprotective

After her younger sister died of leukemia, Kim, 13, felt like all the house rules changed. Suddenly, her mother wouldn't allow her to go to friends' houses or out to the mall. Instead, she was told she needed to stay at home with the family. She complained that her mother was becoming "paranoidly overprotective."

Caleb, 8, had always walked to school. When his father was killed in an automobile accident a block from his house, his mother said he couldn't walk the 10 blocks because it meant passing the accident site and the tree that was scarred from the impact of the accident. When Caleb's mother drove him to school, she also took different streets to avoid the scene. Caleb actually wanted to see the tree.

It's natural for parents to be extra protective of their children after a death, especially if the person who died was another child. A child may want to take a break from activities he or she used to enjoy, or may want to start up sooner than you think. Let the child decide when he or she is ready. Try to remember that connecting with peers and engaging in pleasant activities can be powerful mood boosters for your children. Teens, in particular, find support from peers as well as their family. Participating in activities also helps children see that life, and the things they enjoy in life, can continue even after a loss.

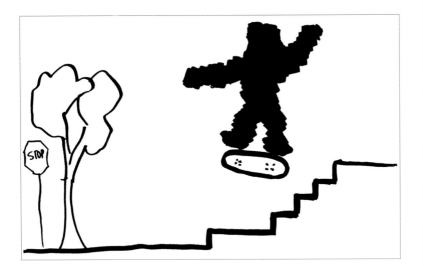

24 Don't force kids to talk

Not all kids are talkers. Often, they express their grief in play, writing or artwork. They may also choose to talk to peers—instead of parents—as trusted confidants. This is especially true of teens, who tend to seek out peers more than their parents for support and friendship. If you are a parent or caregiver, don't be alarmed if a child does not want to talk about grief. And don't assume that a child is not grieving because he or she chooses not to talk. The best approach is to invite and be open to a discussion, while still accepting a child's choice.

Children talk when they are ready and if it helps. In The Dougy Center support groups, children can choose the "I pass" option during the talking circle if they don't want to share. That means they can choose not to speak about a topic the group is discussing. After his dad suicided, Ken, a lanky 14-year-old, attended groups regularly for several months, each time electing to pass in opening circle. One evening, another boy came to the group and shared that his father had died by suicide. When it was his turn, Ken shared his story for the first time. The permission to be silent allowed Ken to take the time he needed to trust the group. He shared his story in his own time.

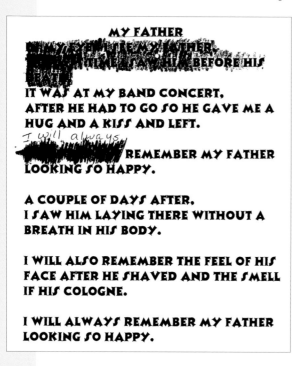

MY FATHER

~~[redacted]~~ BEFORE HIS

IT WAS AT MY BAND CONCERT, AFTER HE HAD TO GO SO HE GAVE ME A HUG AND A KISS AND LEFT.

I will always ~~[redacted]~~ REMEMBER MY FATHER LOOKING SO HAPPY.

A COUPLE OF DAYS AFTER, I SAW HIM LAYING THERE WITHOUT A BREATH IN HIS BODY.

I WILL ALSO REMEMBER THE FEEL OF HIS FACE AFTER HE SHAVED AND THE SMELL IF HIS COLOGNE.

I WILL ALWAYS REMEMBER MY FATHER LOOKING SO HAPPY.

Take a break

Children grieve in cycles. Even when a death is new and parents are grieving intensely, children may be more inclined to play and divert their focus at times from the death. More than adults, they need times to take a break from grief. When possible, plan fun activities for your children that will allow them to let loose, laugh, play and simply be kids.

When Ted, 8, heard about his father's death, the first thing he wanted to do was go out and play. His mother was angry and felt that he didn't show respect for his father. Ted needed to "get out" of the situation because it was too much for him to handle at that moment.

Maryann, 14, and her sister Judy, 12, plan family outings when things feel intense at their house. The sisters go to a funny movie or drive with their mom to their favorite hike by a waterfall. "Sometimes just getting away from the house helps," Maryann says. "It's like catching your breath again."

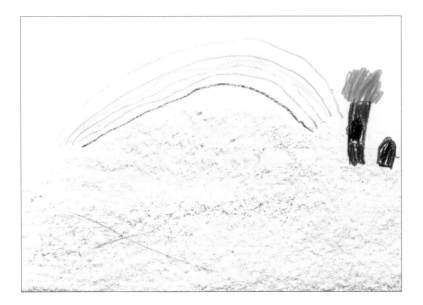

26

Remember: "Playing" is "grieving"

When Jordy was 6, his father died suddenly and unexpectedly of a heroin overdose. Jordy's favorite play activity at The Dougy Center is playing with animals in the sandbox. Once, Jordy chose a small and a large plastic elephant on the toy shelf of the playroom, and brought them over to the sandbox. Clutching the smaller elephant in his fist, he called out, "Daddy, Daddy. Where are you? Where are you?" He dragged the little elephant around the sandbox, then stopped abruptly at the side of the larger elephant. "There he is. There's Dad," Jordy said, in the voice of the little elephant. A look of concern flashed across his face. He squinted. "Uh-oh," he said. "He's dead." Jordy did not continue this story, or begin a conversation about his own father. He picked up his toys and put them back on the shelf.

While adults tend to talk out—or hold in—their grief, a child is more likely to show how he or she feels through play. Very young children don't have the language skills or cognitive development to articulate in words the depths of their emotions. However, they will often use play to enact the struggles in their lives. Children express feelings and thoughts, take on roles of loved ones and tell the stories of their lives in their play. An angry child may not admit to being angry, but will choose to pound on a doll or hit a punching bag. A sad child may draw a picture that represents these feelings. Be sensitive to a grieving child's play. Notice the worlds children create, the roles they take on and the feelings that come up in their play. If you can, reflect back to them what you see and hear, using their words, without any evaluation. This is one way you can validate the experience they are having.

Play

is the natural medium of

expression for children.

Jay's father was sick for more than a year before he died of leukemia. Jay, who often visited his father in the hospital, was 5 when he died. When he visits The Dougy Center, he likes to play doctor. In his play, Jay examines the patients, does surgery and gives medicine to "cure them for good."

Eddie, 5, liked to play with the toy train in The Dougy Center playroom. His mom died of breast cancer. Sometimes, Eddie set up the train track and played for hours. One day, he shared that he and his mom often went down to the train tracks and watched the train go by. "I miss going to see the trains with my mom," he said. Playing with the train brings her memory closer to him.

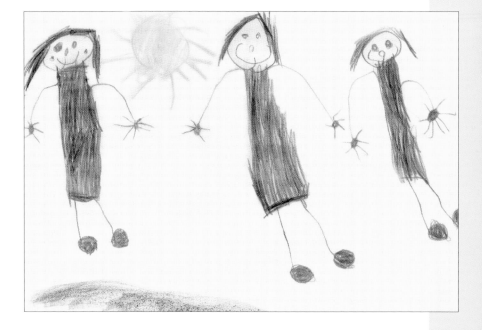

27 Seek additional help for the child if needed

Mild depression, anxiety and behavioral problems are common in children after a death. Grieving children may not feel like eating or may have trouble falling asleep in the initial stages of grief. If physical and emotional symptoms persist and are ongoing, or if they begin to disrupt daily functioning, they should be addressed by a medical professional or a counselor. Some of the signs to watch for include:

- depressed or irritable moods that interfere with healthy living
- loss of interest or pleasure in activities
- sleep disturbances
- appetite increases or decreases
- headaches, stomachaches and other physical symptoms
- fatigue or loss of energy
- thoughts about death, wishing one were dead, suicidal talk
- difficulty concentrating
- social withdrawal

Remember, grieving sometimes looks and feels like depression—especially in the first six months after a death. But a clinically depressed child or teen will usually have at least five symptoms of depression for at least two weeks, and have ongoing difficulty going to school and functioning at home.

Attend to the physical aspects of grief

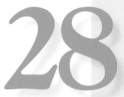

Grief hurts. Sometimes, children experience
physical aches and pains, such as headaches,
stomachaches and other somatic symptoms.
Children also talk about heartaches. Occasionally,
children may complain of pains or tingly sensations
that resemble pains experienced by the parent,
sibling or friend who died. For example, a child whose parent
died of a brain tumor may talk about funny feelings or pains in
his or her head. You may also notice that some grieving children
become more accident prone, falling down and getting bumps and
bruises. Just as we accept and validate emotions, it's important to
do the same for a child's physical concerns. If a child complains of
a stomachache, you might say, "Your stomach is sore and hurting a
lot." Don't assume, of course, that their physical symptoms are all
"in their head." Persistent physical symptoms should be checked
out by a physician.

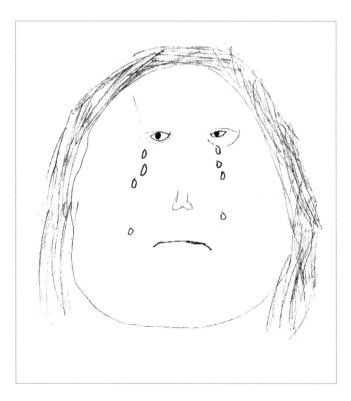

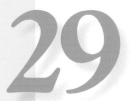

Help children know they are not alone in their grief

Children don't like feeling different from their peers. They don't like to stand out or be left out. They want to belong. When a child no longer has a mom or dad or sibling, he or she is bound to feel awkward when other kids talk about their parents, brothers or sisters. Helping a child find peers who have experienced a death alleviates that sense of being different. Kids are often very relieved to know that they are not the only ones who have had someone close to them die.

Jane, 16, did not want to go to the father-daughter dinner at her high school. Her dad had died the previous summer. Even though her mom tried to encourage Jane to go with her uncle or brother, she refused, saying she would stand out and feel very different. Jenny, a friend, told her, "If your friends are really your friends, they would not treat you any different just because you had a parent die."

For Father's Day, Jeff's fourth-grade teacher asked all the students to make cards for their fathers. Jeff, 9, did not know what to do. His father had died and he felt he couldn't do the activity. Jeff noticed a girl named Katie in his class who was having trouble getting started on her card, so he asked her what she was doing. "My father died when I was 5," Katie said. "So did mine," he replied. Together, the two made pictures remembering activities they enjoyed doing with their dads. Katie drew a picture of herself

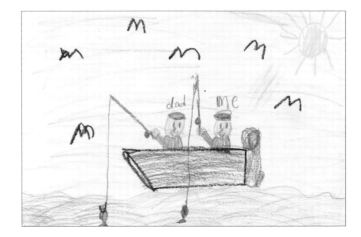

and her dad cooking chocolate chip cookies. Jeff drew a picture of himself and his dad fishing in the river near their home.

Children who have experienced a violent death, such as a suicide or homicide, are particularly vulnerable to feelings of loneliness and isolation. Violent deaths make us nervous because we are not sure what to say or how to react. Typically, when we're uncomfortable our instinct is to withdraw. If you know a child who has experienced a violent death, make an effort to stay in touch and keep the lines of communication open. The child may or may not want to talk about the experience, but he or she needs and depends on loving support from others.

After a violent death, children may have to endure the additional pain of media attention and/or a criminal trial. You might want to call them just to talk. Or, ask if they would like you to accompany them in court. Keep in mind that these children may feel more afraid and vulnerable than they used to. Try to listen to their fears and refrain from evaluating them.

Children who have experienced a suicide death often feel abandoned by the person who died. Sometimes, they feel responsible in some way for the death, or that the suicide reflects poorly on them. They may find it difficult to talk about it, or even to say that someone close to them died by suicide. If you are a teacher, be sensitive to the stigmas that children or others attach to suicide and violent deaths, and help your students to become aware, too.

- Stay in touch. Don't withdraw
- Call during difficult times (e.g. when the media is focusing on the death or when the trial is going on)
- Ask the child if he or she would like to have a friend accompany him or her to the trial or other event
- Be sensitive to stigmas attached to murder, suicide and other violent deaths

30

Understand that grief looks different at different ages

When 5-year-old Nancy saw her deceased father's car in the driveway for the first time since he died, she asked her mother, "Is Daddy home?" Her older sister Kara replied, "Of course not, Daddy died a month ago."

Young children may have difficulty understanding the finality of death. Sometimes, they expect the deceased person to return. They need clear reminders of what it means to be dead. Don't ignore their questions. Little ones also frequently use play as the medium for expressing their grief and remembering aspects of the person who died.

School-age children may ask more detailed questions about the death, and are able to have a more grown-up understanding of what death is. They still tend to "play out," rather than talk through, their feelings around a death. It is also not uncommon for children this age to "act out" in school or in other settings. By acting out, they are trying to get attention. Give it to them. If they don't get the attention they need, they will likely increase the behaviors.

Teens often turn to their peers for support. Given the natural egocentrism that accompanies adolescence, teens may also be wrapped up in their personal emotional response to a death. Teens are focused as well on meaning of life questions, and need to address the "why" questions about a death.

As they mature, children revisit their grief. They may attach a new meaning to the loss or understand it differently. Sometimes, when grief resurfaces years after a death, it catches us off guard and we don't recognize it for what it is. Seventeen-year-old Rita, whose mother died of cancer when she was 6, said she began missing her mom in a new way when she entered high school. "I was feeling sad and lonely. At first I thought it was just because I was in a new school. But I think now it's because I missed having a mom I could share my feelings with," she said. When kids reexperience their grief, adults often worry and want to help them "get over it." A more helpful response is to validate their feelings by listening and supporting them as they work through the change.

Keep in mind, too, that no matter how young children are when someone close dies, they are still impacted by the loss throughout their life span. They may have no memories of the deceased, but they have experienced the loss of someone with whom they shared a significant bond. As members of a family, they are also impacted by the grief of other family members. Finally, they are different from their peers who have not had a death of a parent, sibling or caregiver. Allow them to experience their grief.

For more information on how children grieve at different ages, see the resources guide in the back of this guidebook.

It is diffrent because my baby brother is not there. I fill sad because I fill like it is my falt but I now it is not my falt. My mom feels sad because she looks at my sister and cries because she misses my brother. We go to the mall and watch t.v together. My mom was more sad when my brother Steven died. She is still sad but sometimes now she forgets about it and has a good time.

Me and my mom

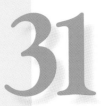

Set limits and rules, and enforce them

In the world of the grieving child, limits and rules are helpful because they help repair the sense of order and structure that was shattered by the death. In the midst of feeling anxious, confused and unsure about what will happen next, it is comforting that some things stay the same. This applies to mealtimes and bedtimes, as well as consequences for breaking rules of the house.

When children are feeling angry or are having difficulty controlling their behavior, continue to enforce household rules. You may feel tempted to make exceptions, but remember it's not helpful to change the rules because it only adds to the chaos and turbulence they are already experiencing. Limits also help provide a safe environment for all members of the family. As you are setting limits, remember you can always validate what a child feels, and can encourage positive and healthy outlets for expressing their emotions.

Setting limits and enforcing rules doesn't mean you shouldn't be flexible when needed—like listening to a child who needs to talk after his or her bedtime. The key here is not rigidity, but providing stability during an unstable time.

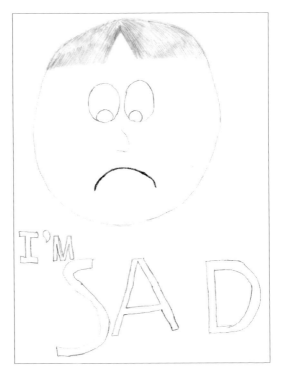

Remember special days that impact the child

Holidays, anniversaries and birthdays are emotional times for everyone. For grievers, holidays can be particularly difficult because they stir up memories of the person who died, re-surfacing feelings of loss. Many grieving families tell us that setting aside time to remember the person who died is helpful on special days.

On the first anniversary of her sister's death from leukemia, Lisa, 14, and her family released a box of butterflies over her grave site.

Marie and her three sons planned a gathering for friends and colleagues on her deceased husband's birthday. "We didn't call it a party," recalls Marie, "but it was a time to celebrate his life. It was important for all of us to take note that before that last terrible act of his life, his suicide, he had given so much to us all. That needed to be remembered, too."

Traditional holidays—Christmas, Yom Kippur, Thanksgiving, Father's Day, Mother's Day—may also be a time to remember the person who died, or to start new family traditions. Invite your children to make creative suggestions on these occasions. Some children may enjoy making a card or lighting a candle for the person who died. What's important is allowing the child to remember the person who died in whatever way he or she chooses.

Plan family times together

Sometimes, it's hard for grieving families to jump back into fun activities they once enjoyed. The absence of the deceased is sharply felt. But families also say it's important to continue to gather and interact both for the sake of the children and for the health of the family unit, because both kids and adults need to have fun.

When a loss is still very new, it may be difficult to find pleasure in things you used to like doing. Or, it may feel like all of you are aware of who is missing. That's normal. Over time, your ability to enjoy activities together will improve.

Jane, 8, and Sam, 6, loved to go camping with their mom and dad. They made it a family affair to pack up the gear and set up the tents. After their dad died, Jane and Sam were afraid they would not ever get to go camping again. Mom decided that it was an important family time, so they got together with another family and went camping as before.

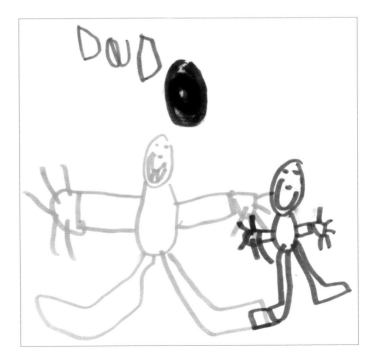

Be available for children when they need you

If you are a parent, your child may need more of your time after a death. Particularly if a child has experienced a parent death, he or she may fear losing you. More than anything, your child needs assurance that you will be there for him or her. Being home when you say you will be is important. Also, provide ways for your children to get in touch with you if they need to reach you.

In sibling deaths, children may feel they are less loved by their parents as they watch their parents grieve over their brother or sister who died. Whenever you can, reassure children of their worth and remind them you love them. A cry for reassurance won't always come when it's convenient. More often than not, it arrives just when you're trying to do something else, such as make it to work on time, drive the car or get dinner on the table. At these moments, even a small, quick reminder of your love helps.

If you are a friend of a grieving child, stay in touch. Even if children don't want to talk, it helps them to know that you are available when they do. Sometimes, grieving children are afraid of burdening their friends with their grief. If you are comfortable listening to and sharing their grief, let them know.

"My aunt is really great. She called me at least once a week to let me talk. She must have big ears. She tells me stuff about my dad when he was a kid."

—Cindy, 13

35 Take care of yourself, and do your own grieving

Children take cues from their parents and other adults around them. If you are doing your own grief work in whatever way is healthy for you, your child will be more likely to do the same. In households where parents hide their grief, children are likely to follow suit. Also, doing your own work allows you to be more present and available for your child, even in the midst of sadness and loss. If you are taking care of yourself, you will have more energy to give your children and will be less likely to vent your frustrations on them.

"My dad got really depressed. Our priest told him about some psychologist. He's a lot better now. I don't know what they did, but he's more normal again."

—James, 15

"My mom started drinking again after my sister died. She stopped going to AA. I'm afraid she's alcoholic again. She really needs help. I think my parents are about ready to get a divorce."

—Craig, 11

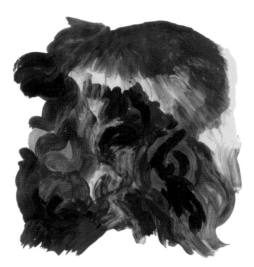

Resources

Also by The Dougy Center for Grieving Children

More in our Guidebook Series:

- **Helping Children Cope with Death**

   This guidebook offers a comprehensive, easy-to-read overview of how children grieve and strategies to support them. Based on The Dougy Center's work with thousands of grieving children and their families, you will learn how children understand death, how to talk with children about death at various developmental stages, how to be helpful and when to seek outside help. This book is useful for parents, teachers, helping professionals and anyone trying to support a grieving child.

- **Helping the Grieving Student: A Guide for Teachers**

   At some point, every teacher will encounter a student who has been affected by a death. This guidebook is an essential resource for elementary-, middle- and high-school teachers, offering practical tips and information for how to respond to a death.

- **When Death Impacts Your School: A Guide for School Administrators**

   This is a valuable resource for school personnel who are faced with a death or tragedy in their school community. This guidebook includes suggestions for how schools can help students—by addressing concerns, organizing memorials and offering support. It also includes instructions for developing a school intervention plan after a death, how to address issues related to suicide and violence and how to decide when outside help is needed.

- **Helping Teens Cope with Death**

   This practical guide covers the unique grief responses of teenagers and the specific challenges they face when grieving a death. You will learn how death impacts teenagers and ways that you can help them. The book also offers advice from parents and caregivers of bereaved teens on how to support adolescents and how to determine when professional help is needed.

- **What About the Kids? Understanding Their Needs in Funeral Planning and Services**

  This book addresses the best practices for funeral and memorial services with children and teens. Learn how to include children in these rituals and creative ways to involve them in the process. You will find suggestions from children and teens about what was helpful and unhelpful about the funeral or memorial service they attended.

- **Waving Goodbye: An Activity Manual for Children in Grief**

  Waving Goodbye features more than 45 activities to use with children and teens in peer support groups or for parents to use with their children. These activities are categorized by topic and are designed to help children process their unique grief.

- **After a Suicide: A Workbook for Grieving Kids**

  In this hands-on, interactive workbook, children who have been exposed to a suicide can learn from other grieving kids. The workbook includes drawing activities, puzzles, stories, advice from other kids and helpful suggestions for how to navigate the grief process after a suicide death.

- **After a Murder: A Workbook for Grieving Kids**

  Through the stories, thoughts and feelings of other kids who have experienced a murder, this hands-on workbook allows children to see that they are not alone in their feelings and experiences. The workbook includes drawing activities, puzzles and word games to help explain confusing elements specific to a murder, such as the police, media and legal system.

The above resources can be ordered through:
The Dougy Center
P.O. Box 86852
Portland, OR 97286
503-775-5683
Fax: 503-777-3097
Website: www.dougy.org

What is The Dougy Center?

The mission of The Dougy Center is to provide loving support in a safe place where children, teens and their families who are grieving a death can share their experiences as they move through their healing processes. Through our National Center for Grieving Children & Families, we also provide support and training locally, nationally and internationally to individuals and organizations seeking to assist children and teens in grief.

The Dougy Center serves children and teens, ages 3 to 19, who have experienced the death of a parent or sibling (or, in our teen groups, a friend), to accident, illness, suicide or murder. The support groups are coordinated by professional staff and trained volunteers. In addition, the parents or caregivers of the youth participate in support groups to address their needs and the issues of raising children following a traumatic loss.

When The Dougy Center was established in 1982, it was the first grief peer support program of its kind in the country. In response to numerous requests for information about our program, The Dougy Center has developed trainings and publications to help other communities establish centers for grieving children and families. Through our National Center for Grieving Children, The Dougy Center has trained individuals and groups throughout the world and publishes a National Directory of Children's Grief Services, updated annually.

The Dougy Center is a 501(c)3 nonprofit organization and raises its entire budget through contributions from individuals, businesses and foundations. We receive no federal funding or third-party payments. Participating families may contribute to the program, but there is no fee for service. While families receiving services contribute what they can, many do not have the financial resources to donate. Because The Center never turns a family away because of their inability to contribute, we are completely reliant upon private support from our friends in the community.

How can I support The Dougy Center or get additional information about its programs?

Contributions to The Dougy Center are tax-deductible to the full extent allowable under IRS guidelines. Your gift can be made out to The Dougy Center and mailed to us at the address below.

You can also receive additional information about:

- other guidebooks available from The Dougy Center
- videos and other resource materials available from The Dougy Center
- training for developing a children's grief center in your area
- the National Summer Institute held annually at The Dougy Center on developing a children's grief center in your area
- how to schedule a training or presentation in your area
- supporting The Dougy Center and its local and national programs to assist grieving children through a will or bequest

Write, call, fax or email:

The Dougy Center
P.O. Box 86852
Portland, OR 97286

503-775-5683
Fax: 503-777-3097

Email: help@dougy.org
Website: www.dougy.org

The Dougy Center
could not exist without
the generous contributions
of hundreds of volunteers,
who give of their time, boundless energy,
unflagging enthusiasm and matchless dedication.
We thank them for accompanying
the children, teens and adults
who come to The Dougy Center
in their grief journeys.

Notes

Notes